Welcome.

This journey is yours.

So here is a record, unique to you.

Create your plan, set your goals, track your progress...

And enjoy the journey!

Training can be fun. However, always put safety first, and always inspect your training space for obstacles and hazards upon entry. Also, inspect your apparatus before every training session. For Pole- is it stable and secure? Does it need a clean? For Aerials, inspect your fabrics, your ropes, are they still intact, with nothing spilt on them or frayed, no rips or holes? What about your rigging? It should have been set up by a qualified rigger. But check your equipment, are your karabiners still gravity loaded? Are they done up? *Please do not play with or touch any hardware or rigging if this is not your qualification base. But it is important to check (eye-ball) these things for your own safety and peace of mind.

Disclaimer:

I'm a pole fitness instructor and not a healthcare professional. This book only provides general information about pole fitness and does not consider your personal circumstances in any way. Circus Aerials and Pole Fitness are high-risk sports. You should consult your health care professional before starting any fitness program to ensure that it is right for your needs and abilities. Do not start a pole fitness or aerial program if your pole fitness instructor or health care provider advises against it. Please monitor and work within your own limitations, and stop immediately if you experience things like faintness, dizziness, pain, or even shortness of breath at any time while exercising. Remember that your body needs to rest. Training regimes need to allow for rest and recovery as well. This manual is not a substitute for skilled instruction. We recommend seeking professional instruction from a pole fitness instructor before attempting a pole fitness program on your own, always having a competent individual close by to assist if needed. Please ensure that your pole set-up and area is secure, safe, and as per manufacturers specifications, ensuring an unobstructed space. To the extent permitted by law, I disclaim any liability (including negligence) arising directly or indirectly from your use of this manual or any of the information contained in this book.

Second Edition April 2022

Pole Moves

Inspirations

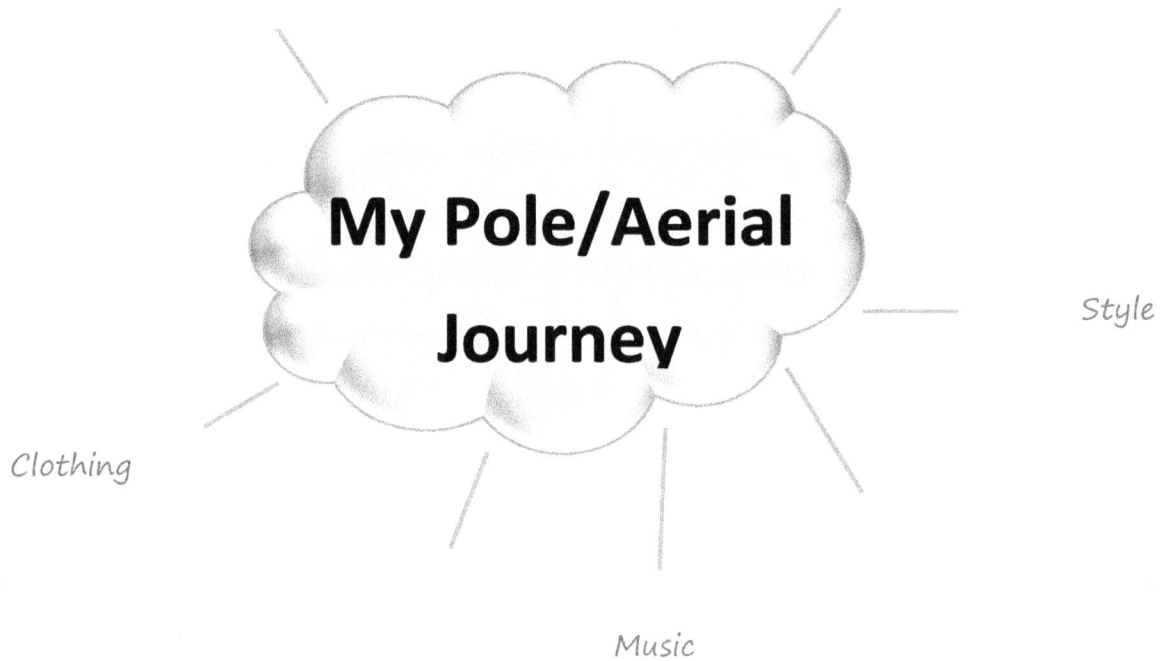

My Pole/Aerial Journey

Style

Clothing

Music

How I want to feel

Where I want to pole

My Ultimate Goal:

_____

_____

_____

_____

How it looks/Describe it:

(This could be any product of your goal, if your goal is a confidence boost, how does that look as you walk down the street, or present yourself etc.)

_____

_____

_____

<table>
<tr><td colspan="2">Your Goal Should be SMART:</td></tr>
<tr><td colspan="2">**Specific**, (and simple)</td></tr>
<tr><td colspan="2">**Measurable**, (know when it is done)</td></tr>
<tr><td colspan="2">**Achievable**, (can the big goal be divided into little goal steps?)</td></tr>
<tr><td colspan="2">**Realistic**, and</td></tr>
<tr><td colspan="2">**Timely** (manageable time frame - too long is off putting!)</td></tr>
</table>

What it makes me feel like:

_____

_____

_____

_____

Steps to achieve that goal:

Steps (mini-goals)	Achieved by (date)	Completed date

If you pursue your dreams, then they can come true.

Why create a Vision Board?

- ✓ Be able to visualise your goal - Seeing is believing!
- ✓ Increases your motivation, focus, productivity, and determination!
- ✓ Increases your chance of success!
- ✓ Clarifies what you want and makes the dream real in your mind
- ✓ Creates an emotional connection which helps with motivation

There is no definite "starting point" – begin wherever feels right for you.

How to create a Vision board?

- ✓ Think about your goals- the big questions, think about them, and break them down.
  - o What activities, style, moves do you want to learn
  - o Is there something you want to get better at? Straight lines, pointed toes, deadlifting strength? – what makes this move feel right to you?
  - o What is the next step? Is it a personal goal, a career goal, or a perfect move for a photoshoot?
- ✓ Believe in your goals and yourself!
- ✓ What is your theme now you have broken down your goals and aims? Is it particular to a move, or an event coming up, is it a style of movement? -now decide, do you want a very specific mood/vision board, or a more theme-based generalised one reflecting a style or a flow or even a look.
- ✓ Now start creating... pick your style or format... find images, photos, colours, words of inspiration. Keep it all positive and get creative with the scissors and glue!

Don't just talk about it, that isn't starting.
Quit the talk and get started!

My Vision Board

Woohoo... This is me!!

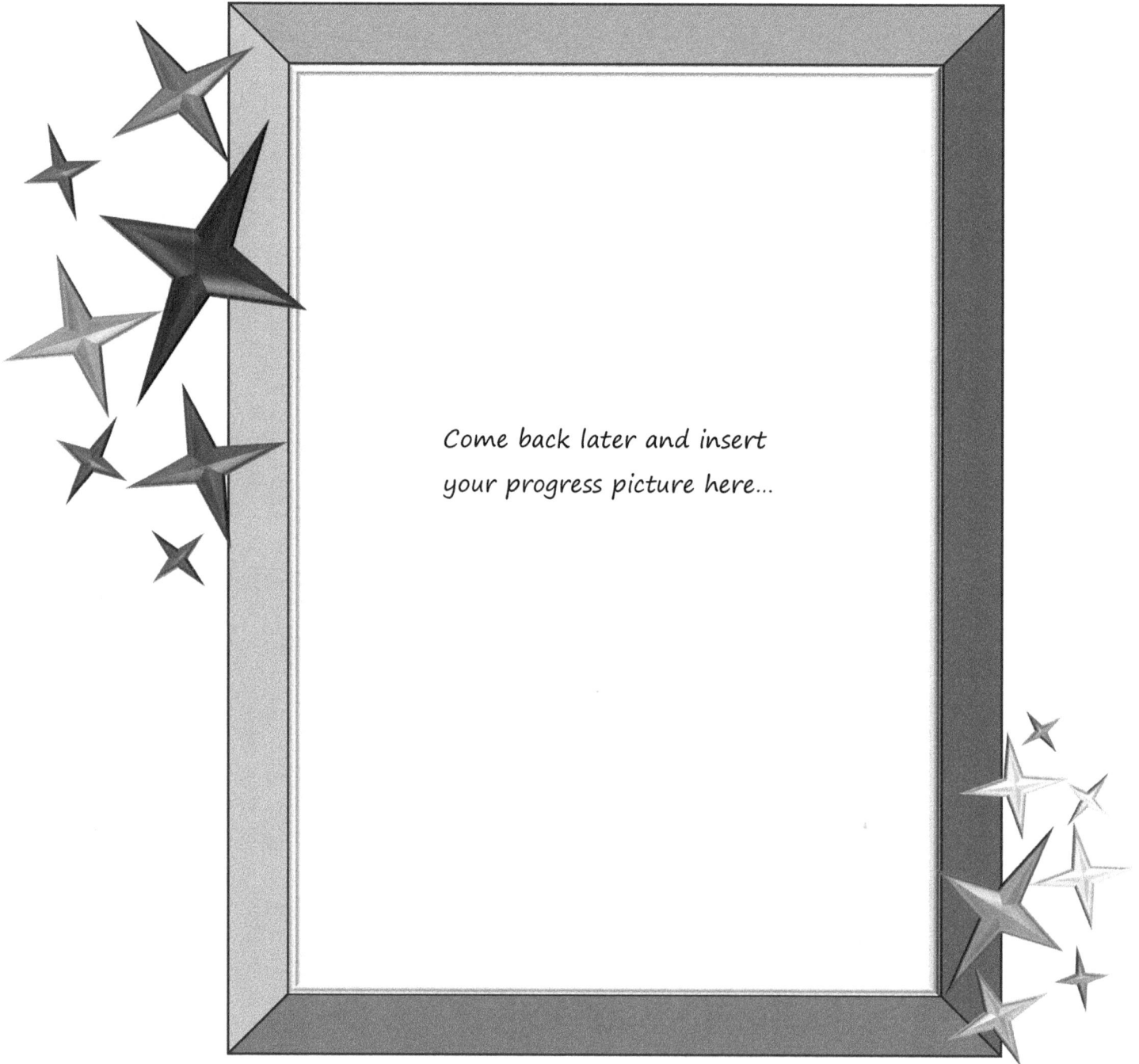

Come back later and insert
your progress picture here...

Having achieved my goal, I feel....

_____

_____

_____

_____

You are unique! The more you that you are, the less like someone else you are. Logical
right? So be you! Do your journey! Be unique! ... An artist like no other!

Important Things to remember on your journey:

- ✓ Always warm-up and cool-down!
- ✓ Use your Wings (lift through your lower trapezius muscle) – I roll my shoulders back before each move as a cue to not hang out of my shoulders, instead lifting with my wings.
- ✓ Remember to pull and push in your grips on the pole.
- ✓ Keep hydrated! (With water!)
- ✓ Finish your moves nicely (create good safe habits)
- ✓ Breathe!!
- ✓ If on the pole- Your pushing arm is straight, it should be exactly that, straight- be careful if there is a hyperextension in your elbow, work on low-risk moves to strengthen muscles to keep it straight.
- ✓ You will have a "training face" – what face do you always pull for your movies and photos? Being aware of it is step 1... step 2, either smile, relax, pick a character or an emotion, and play with dancing in different ways to relax your "training concentration face."
- ✓ Where is your random floating hand- give it a job, a purpose... don't let it detract from your moves.
- ✓ Point your toes- or if they are flexed, it should be purposeful and part of the act.
- ✓ Work within your limits and always listen to your body. Pole Fitness and Aerials are high risk. Only perform moves you are ready for, and if you are fatiguing, listen to your body and adjust the session. I normally end up with a splits training session when I am fatigued. Alternatively, I add in floor conditioning for the move I was working on; if my body will allow it.
- ✓ Allow yourself time to rest and recover.
- ✓ Have fun!!! – that is what this is all about.

Need some examples?!

Here are some of the older format that have been filled out in the past...

Beginner Level....

Use your own cue's and words to help you remember and understand!

Personal Pole Record

Date: 1 December 2020   Level: Begnners (Level 1)

Getting Started (10min)

Cardio Warm Up
- boxing sequence
- slowed to flowy circular hip circles, chest circles, body rolls, liquid flow

Dynamic Stretches
- high kicks
- wrist, elbow & arm circles
- chest openers
- neck semi circles
- hip openers

Conditioning
- the pull up onto tippy toes x3
- push up on knees

Core Moves to work on today

Move Name: (sketch if needed)	Move Name: (sketch if needed)	Move Name: (sketch if needed)
fireman spin	front knee hook	back knee hook
Prep Move 1: false step around/ step around (or dip spin)	**Prep Move 1:** basic spin grip (- fireman spin)	**Prep Move 1:** *front knee hook → but go back after going back as hip alignment clicks.
Prep Move 2: step through move placement before adding momentum to spin	**Prep Move 2:** - step through move bringing it to the floor for extra 2 secs of conditioning.	**Prep Move 2:** reverse/ backwards spin grip
- basic spin grip - outside leg in front, knee to one side, foot to other - Push off tapping inside leg to back of pole, knee to free side, foot to other	- basic spin grip - bend inside leg onto pole at comfortable height - up onto tippy toe - lean forward thru hips - bend knees.	

Choreography Notes
1st combo- Fireman into back
Practice walking/flowing in
- walk crossing your foot ove

Cool Down and Stretch (10m
- All chest/shoulder/back st & quads, glutes & neck.

Personal Pole Record

Self-Evaluation

Notes to improve and work on next time
- not lifting into spins. letting gravity help
- hips forward in knee hooks!

Tricky move: Front knees. **Muscles/muscle groups to work on:** ham strings, (stretch hip flexors) lower traps & shoulder/rotator cuff muscles

What tips helped me today

Move Name:	Move Name:	Other:
Fireman spin	Front knee hook.	Back knee hook
- Place legs, don't jump. - It's okay to hold on like crazy at first! learn to trust your grip.	- Santa belly. - lean forwards through the hips until gravity takes you around.	- wait until calf touches before bending knee - Palm faces direction you are going

Something that really clicked with me today
the grip! - I can hold myself and its ok to slide!

Favourite or Inspiring Music Track
moves like Jagger
& Don't stop believin'

My goal (something I am looking forward to)
being able to put two spins together

♡ I am proud of myself because...
I tried even though I had my doubts and may have more stregnth than I thought.

Personal Pole Record

Date: 22 Jan 2021   **Level:** Intermediate (Level 2)

Getting Started (10min)

Cardio Warm Up	Dynamic Stretches	Conditioning
- squat kicks (kick in them) - high knees jog - embody an animal walking along hot coals.	- wrist, elbows, arm circles. - washing machine arms - chest & hip circles - hip openers - chest openers - high side kicks	- basic invert grip, hips infront, lift one knee up, hold & snap legs over. - Pole lifts & hold. - Push ups - bicycle crunches - oblique crunches

Core Moves to work on today

Move Name: (sketch if needed)	Move Name: (sketch if needed)	Move Name: (sketch if needed)
Cradle variation (straightening top leg)	Carousel kick	Pole sit.
Prep Move 1: basic cradle.	**Prep Move 1:** Pole lifts	**Prep Move 1:** hold pole chest height, squat down, slide pole until its at upper thigh. Cross one leg on top, lean to that side. take foot off floor
Prep Move 2: bow & arrow hold. (Cradle grip, point top toe to ceiling)	**Prep Move 2:** Fireman to pole stand.	**Prep Move 2:** no hand prep - standing, hook inside leg, behind pole, foot in front. bring torso infront arms
- outside arm shoulder height, inside arm down, 45° to pole. - chest across. - legs up to cradle, inside leg first. - straighten top leg, knees together	- knee to one side, foot to other, all of shin on pole. - same top to p leg - Push in a rocket ba	- hold chest height (stabilize not lift)

Choreogr

- slow placement...cra fold it back in to cro
- play with transitions in

Cool Down and

- All chest/shoulder/bac Quads, obliques
- rotate moving through liquid, flowing to

Personal Pole Record

Self-Evaluation

Notes to improve and work on next time

Lifting in to pole sit.
Smoothing out my dismounts.

Tricky move: cradle   **Muscles/muscle groups to work on:**
Bicep. & Abs.
Stretch & strengthen obliques.

What tips helped me today

Move Name: Sit.	Move Name: carousel kick	Other: cradle variation
- tilt top leg/hip towards the pole → pinchy!! - pain does desensitize!! ~6ish weeks.	- shoot torso up like a rocket ship - top leg - knee at hip height. Push into pole.	- don't rush, slow down placement - tilt/tip down into it

Something that really clicked with me today

getting my chest infront with a sit!!

Favourite or Inspiring Music Track

Greatest Showman → This is me.

My goal (something I am looking forward to)

- being able to use carousel kick to get into moves up the pole.
- Pole climb!

♡ I am proud of myself because...
even though it was pinchy, I still did a pole sit!

Level: _____   Date: _____

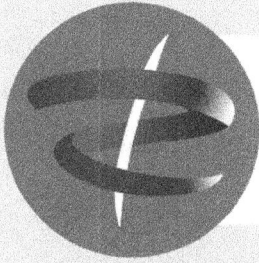

Training Record

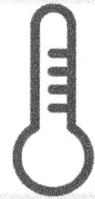

Colour in how stressed you are

Getting Started (10min)

Cardio Warm up:

Dynamic Stretches:

Conditioning:

Core Moves to work on today

Move Name:

Draw/sketch:

Prep Move 1:

Prep Move 2:

Notes:

Move Name:

Draw/sketch:

Prep Move 1:

Prep Move 2:

Notes:

Move Name:

Draw/sketch:

Prep Move 1:

Prep Move 2:

Notes:

Choreography notes

Cool down and stretch (10 min)

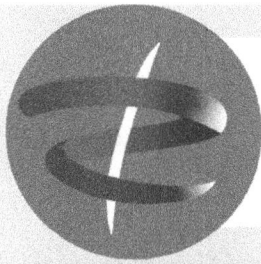

Self- Evaluation

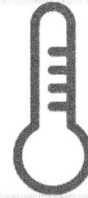

Notes to improve on next time

Tricky move and the muscle groups to work on

Move Name: _____

Strengthen:

Stretch:

Other notes:

What tips helped me today?

Move Name: _____

Move Name: _____

Other: _____

Something that really clicked with me

Favourite or Inspiring music track

My Goal (something I look forward to)

I am proud of myself because...

Level: Date:

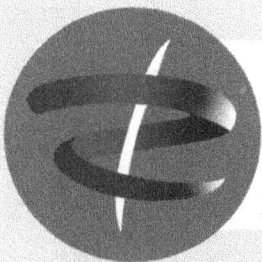

Training Record

Colour in how stressed you are

Getting Started (10min)

Cardio Warm up:

Dynamic Stretches:

Conditioning:

Core Moves to work on today

Move Name:

Draw/sketch:

Prep Move 1:

Prep Move 2:

Notes:

Move Name:

Draw/sketch:

Prep Move 1:

Prep Move 2:

Notes:

Move Name:

Draw/sketch:

Prep Move 1:

Prep Move 2:

Notes:

Choreography notes

Cool down and stretch (10 min)

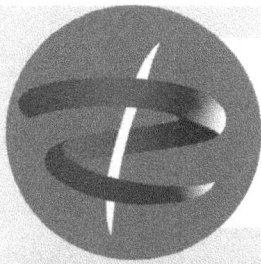

Self- Evaluation

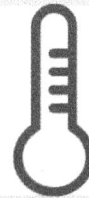

Notes to improve on next time

Tricky move and the muscle groups to work on

Move Name: _____

Strengthen:

Stretch:

Other notes:

What tips helped me today?

Move Name: _____

Move Name: _____

Other: _____

Something that really clicked with me

Favourite or Inspiring music track

My Goal (something I look forward to)

I am proud of myself because...

Level: _____   Date: _____

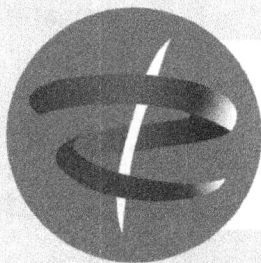

Training Record

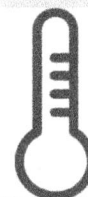

Colour in
how
stressed
you are

Getting Started (10min)

Cardio Warm up:

Dynamic Stretches:

Conditioning:

Core Moves to work on today

Move Name:
Draw/sketch:

Prep Move 1:

Prep Move 2:

Notes:

Move Name:
Draw/sketch:

Prep Move 1:

Prep Move 2:

Notes:

Move Name:
Draw/sketch:

Prep Move 1:

Prep Move 2:

Notes:

Choreography notes

Cool down and stretch (10 min)

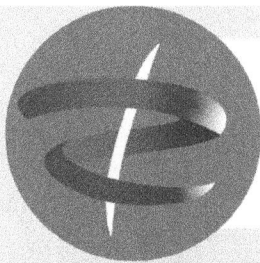

Self- Evaluation

Colour in how fatigued you are

Notes to improve on next time

Tricky move and the muscle groups to work on

Move Name: _____

Strengthen:

Stretch:

Other notes:

What tips helped me today?

Move Name: _____

Move Name: _____

Other: _____

Something that really clicked with me

Favourite or Inspiring music track

My Goal (something I look forward to)

I am proud of myself because...

Level: _____   Date: _____

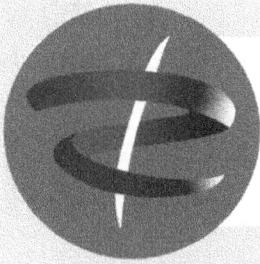

Training Record

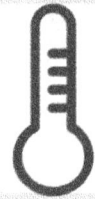

Getting Started (10min)

Cardio Warm up:

Dynamic Stretches:

Conditioning:

Core Moves to work on today

Move Name:

Draw/sketch:

Prep Move 1:

Prep Move 2:

Notes:

Move Name:

Draw/sketch:

Prep Move 1:

Prep Move 2:

Notes:

Move Name:

Draw/sketch:

Prep Move 1:

Prep Move 2:

Notes:

Choreography notes

Cool down and stretch (10 min)

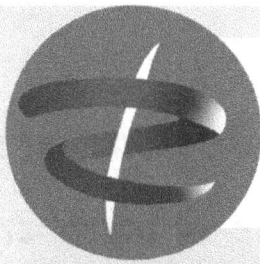

Self- Evaluation

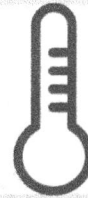

Notes to improve on next time

Tricky move and the muscle groups to work on

Move Name: _____

Strengthen:

Stretch:

Other notes:

What tips helped me today?

Move Name: _____

Move Name: _____

Other: _____

Something that really clicked with me

Favourite or Inspiring music track

My Goal (something I look forward to)

I am proud of myself because...

Your mind and body won't progress in your art if you don't allow it time to rest. Rest is vital to your continual progress.

Signs that you need rest:

- You feel like you are always tired.
- You feel sick after the warm-up.
- You feel like you aren't on top of things and keeping up with your usual tasks.
- Stress and anxiety feel like they are creeping up on you, sometimes making it harder to sleep and unable to rest.
- You're sore- more often and for longer, like even after 2-3 days- Everything aches, old ailments are niggling you.
- Your cranky, angry, and easily irritated (I get emotional and upset! My hubby gets headaches and anxiety.)
- Cracked lips- Michael J. Breus, PhD — expert in sleep disorders, has said that dry lips are a sign of dehydration, which can affect sleeping patterns and bodily functions.
- Transitions and lines in your training are looking sloppy- quality of movement has deteriorated- You feel like you're not making any progress.
- Drinking water isn't making you feel hydrated.
- Your normal tricks and combinations aren't working for you as easily as they should, they feel heavy and messy... your bendy tricks, less-bendy, your strength tricks need so much more effort.
- You pressed snooze countless times on your alarm and, you're still tired!

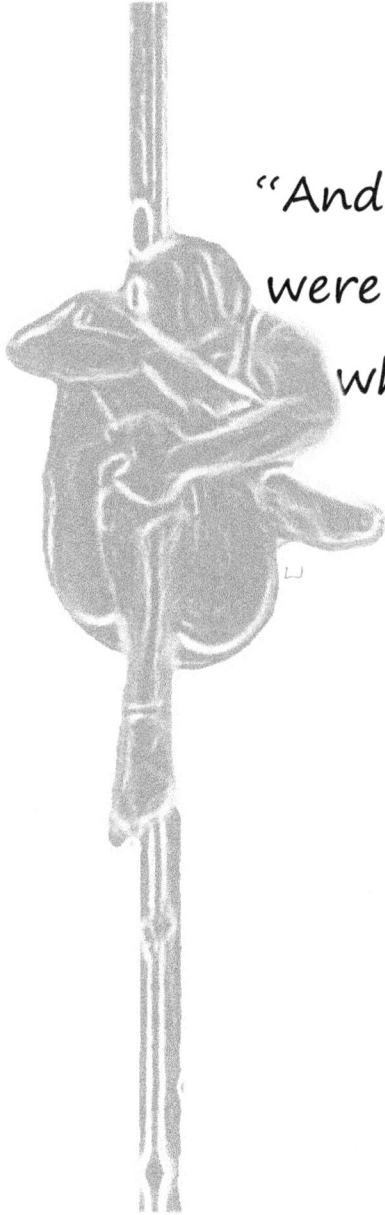

"And those who were seen dancing,
were thought to be insane by those
who couldn't hear the music"

–Friedrich Nietzsche

Level: _____   Date: _____

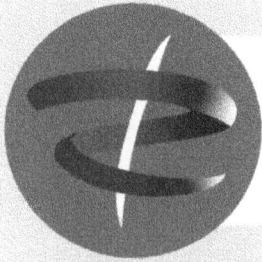

Training Record

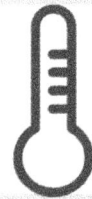

Getting Started (10min)

Cardio Warm up:

Dynamic Stretches:

Conditioning:

Core Moves to work on today

Move Name:

Draw/sketch:

Prep Move 1:

Prep Move 2:

Notes:

Move Name:

Draw/sketch:

Prep Move 1:

Prep Move 2:

Notes:

Move Name:

Draw/sketch:

Prep Move 1:

Prep Move 2:

Notes:

Choreography notes

Cool down and stretch (10 min)

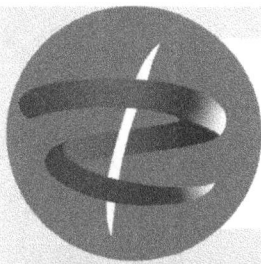

Self- Evaluation

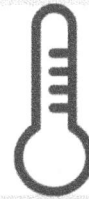

Colour in how fatigued you are

Notes to improve on next time

Tricky move and the muscle groups to work on

Move Name: _____

Strengthen:

Stretch:

Other notes:

What tips helped me today?

Move Name: _____

Move Name: _____

Other: _____

Something that really clicked with me

Favourite or Inspiring music track

My Goal (something I look forward to)

I am proud of myself because...

Level:

Date:

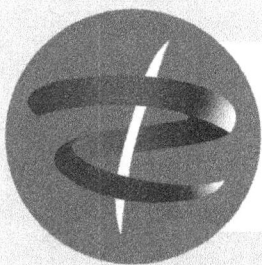

Training Record

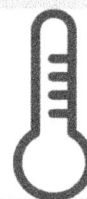

Colour in how stressed you are

Getting Started (10min)

Cardio Warm up:

Dynamic Stretches:

Conditioning:

Core Moves to work on today

Move Name:

Draw/sketch:

Prep Move 1:

Prep Move 2:

Notes:

Move Name:

Draw/sketch:

Prep Move 1:

Prep Move 2:

Notes:

Move Name:

Draw/sketch:

Prep Move 1:

Prep Move 2:

Notes:

Choreography notes

Cool down and stretch (10 min)

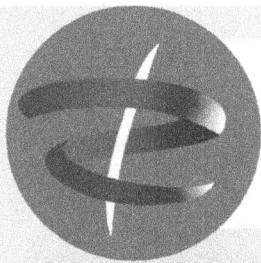

Self- Evaluation

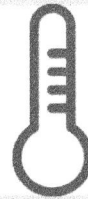

Colour in how fatigued you are

Notes to improve on next time

Tricky move and the muscle groups to work on

Move Name: _____

Strengthen:

Stretch:

Other notes:

What tips helped me today?

Move Name: _____

Move Name: _____

Other: _____

Something that really clicked with me

Favourite or Inspiring music track

My Goal (something I look forward to)

I am proud of myself because...

Level: _____   Date: _____

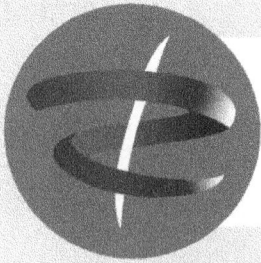

Training Record

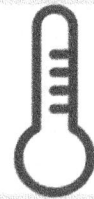

Colour in how stressed you are

Getting Started (10min)

Cardio Warm up:

Dynamic Stretches:

Conditioning:

Core Moves to work on today

Move Name:

Draw/sketch:

Prep Move 1:

Prep Move 2:

Notes:

Move Name:

Draw/sketch:

Prep Move 1:

Prep Move 2:

Notes:

Move Name:

Draw/sketch:

Prep Move 1:

Prep Move 2:

Notes:

Choreography notes

Cool down and stretch (10 min)

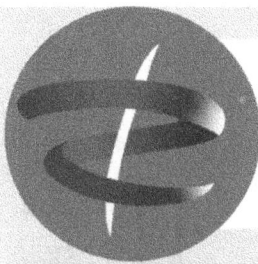

Self- Evaluation

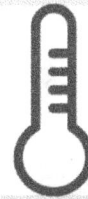

Notes to improve on next time

Tricky move and the muscle groups to work on

Move Name: _____

Strengthen:

Stretch:

Other notes:

What tips helped me today?

Move Name: _____

Move Name: _____

Other: _____

Something that really clicked with me

Favourite or Inspiring music track

My Goal (something I look forward to)

I am proud of myself because...

Level: _____   Date: _____

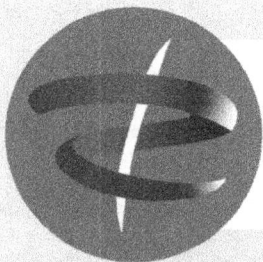

Training Record

Colour in how stressed you are

Getting Started (10min)

Cardio Warm up:

Dynamic Stretches:

Conditioning:

Core Moves to work on today

Move Name:

Draw/sketch:

Prep Move 1:

Prep Move 2:

Notes:

Move Name:

Draw/sketch:

Prep Move 1:

Prep Move 2:

Notes:

Move Name:

Draw/sketch:

Prep Move 1:

Prep Move 2:

Notes:

Choreography notes

Cool down and stretch (10 min)

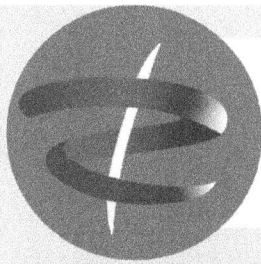

Self- Evaluation

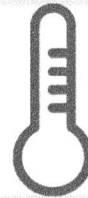

Notes to improve on next time

Tricky move and the muscle groups to work on

Move Name: _____

Strengthen:

Stretch:

Other notes:

What tips helped me today?

Move Name: _____

Move Name: _____

Other: _____

Something that really clicked with me

Favourite or Inspiring music track

My Goal (something I look forward to)

I am proud of myself because...

Remember, to master something, you need to practice, learn, and grow. This comes from failing, again and again. Don't be disheartened as a beginner, you are on your way to mastery.

Celebrate your success!

I am Proud of this move...

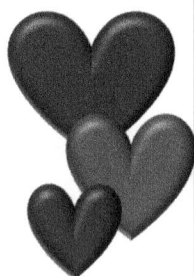

Insert your picture here...

Pictures are so universal, 1000 words they say, but it is a method that has no language barrier. Arguably, the most effective method of communication.

Good Habits

1. Do something, even if it is a stretch day, or a floor workday, don't just push the training day a side.

2. Make it social, share your goals, your progress, and even your mishaps

3. Always prepare, get everything ready, know what you want to do (even if it is a freestyle session, know that is your plan)

4. Practice the dodgy side! It is important to always keep your body balanced, even starting your training session on your bad side, as you spend more time on the first side you train. So, once you have a move, the next time you go to train it, give the dodgy side a go first.

5. Practice new skills, first- before you fatigue! (After your warm-up of course) New skills require more thought and thus tire you out more.

6. Keep it Fun, mix it up, and make it interesting.

7. Practice the stuff you aren't good at! You know how you find a move, it's really hard, or bitey, and you leave it be. Done it once, won't do it again! No... go on... do it... practice! Safely of course! Let yourself move past this barrier, let your mind and body grow beyond it.

8. Think Positive. Celebrate the little wins. Negative self-talk is unhealthy, but having a positive internal dialogue is fantastic. Keep it progress-focused and see how much better you feel about your training.

9. Remember there is always more to learn! Curiosity, enthusiasm and the expectation to learn are stepping stones to growth. No one knows everything, be prepared to learn from mistakes, and never stop learning.

10. Self-Analysis- take a photo, or a video, have a look, what do you like, what do you need to work on? Being critical of your own moves can be very hard, but if you can see the positives and the points you need to work on it is amazing for your growth!

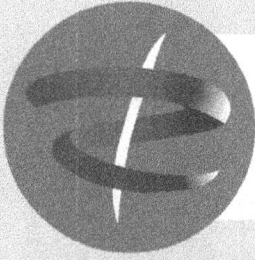

Flexibility Goals

What it will look like when I have achieved my goal.

Muscles required to condition or stretch for this to happen?

Stretch:

Strengthen:

Flexibility and conditioning drills, reps and requirements

Remember to maintain balance, remember you have a right and left side, as well as front and back. balance your training, not only in your body, but in relation to strength and flexibility.

Time Frame

Training how many days a week:

For how long?

Goal is to by achieved by:

Mini Goals that help with my big goal

Things I need to be able to achieve to reach my goal:

Notes

What days per week do I do this?   Level:

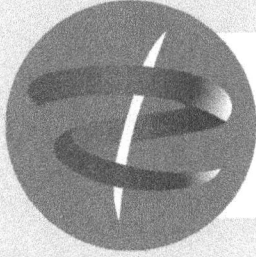

Flexibility Workout Planner

Warm Up

Training Drill (strength or flex)

Time

How long do I stretch this for?

Remember, it is not just about flexibility, it is also about ensuring your muscles are strong enough to maintain the flexibility without causing issues.

Cool Down

Level: Date:

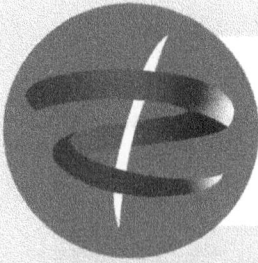

Training Record

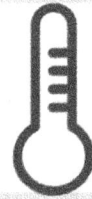

Colour in how stressed you are

Getting Started (10min)

Cardio Warm up:

Dynamic Stretches:

Conditioning:

Core Moves to work on today

Move Name:

Draw/sketch:

Prep Move 1:

Prep Move 2:

Notes:

Move Name:

Draw/sketch:

Prep Move 1:

Prep Move 2:

Notes:

Move Name:

Draw/sketch:

Prep Move 1:

Prep Move 2:

Notes:

Choreography notes

Cool down and stretch (10 min)

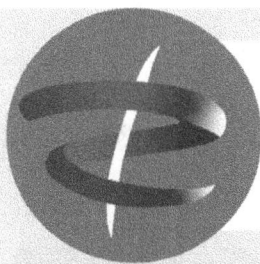

Self- Evaluation

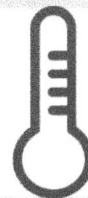

Notes to improve on next time

Tricky move and the muscle groups to work on

Move Name: _____

Strengthen:

Stretch:

Other notes:

What tips helped me today?

Move Name: _____

Move Name: _____

Other: _____

Something that really clicked with me

Favourite or Inspiring music track

My Goal (something I look forward to)

I am proud of myself because...

Level: Date:

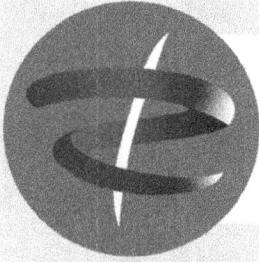

Training Record

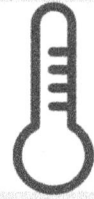

Colour in how stressed you are

Getting Started (10min)

Cardio Warm up:

Dynamic Stretches:

Conditioning:

Core Moves to work on today

Move Name:

Draw/sketch:

Prep Move 1:

Prep Move 2:

Notes:

Move Name:

Draw/sketch:

Prep Move 1:

Prep Move 2:

Notes:

Move Name:

Draw/sketch:

Prep Move 1:

Prep Move 2:

Notes:

Choreography notes

Cool down and stretch (10 min)

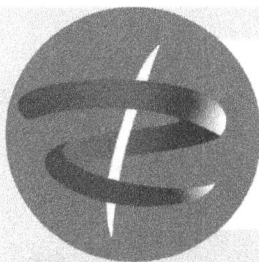

Self- Evaluation

Colour in how fatigued you are

Notes to improve on next time

Tricky move and the muscle groups to work on

Move Name: _____

Strengthen:

Stretch:

Other notes:

What tips helped me today?

Move Name: _____

Move Name: _____

Other: _____

Something that really clicked with me

Favourite or Inspiring music track

My Goal (something I look forward to)

I am proud of myself because...

Level: Date:

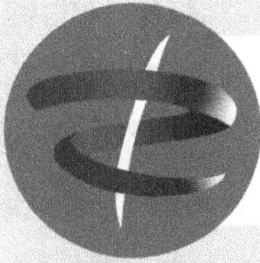

Training Record

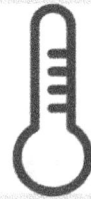

Colour in how stressed you are

Getting Started (10min)

Cardio Warm up:

Dynamic Stretches:

Conditioning:

Core Moves to work on today

Move Name:

Draw/sketch:

Prep Move 1:

Prep Move 2:

Notes:

Move Name:

Draw/sketch:

Prep Move 1:

Prep Move 2:

Notes:

Move Name:

Draw/sketch:

Prep Move 1:

Prep Move 2:

Notes:

Choreography notes

Cool down and stretch (10 min)

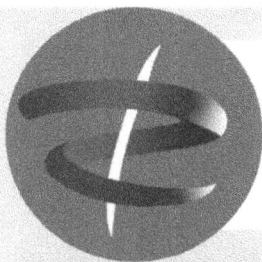

Self- Evaluation

Notes to improve on next time

Tricky move and the muscle groups to work on

Move Name: _____

Strengthen:

Stretch:

Other notes:

What tips helped me today?

Move Name: _____

Move Name: _____

Other: _____

Something that really clicked with me

Favourite or Inspiring music track

My Goal (something I look forward to)

I am proud of myself because...

Level: Date:

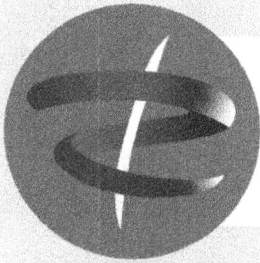

Training Record

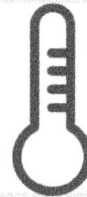

Colour in how stressed you are

Getting Started (10min)

Cardio Warm up:

Dynamic Stretches:

Conditioning:

Core Moves to work on today

Move Name:

Draw/sketch:

Prep Move 1:

Prep Move 2:

Notes:

Move Name:

Draw/sketch:

Prep Move 1:

Prep Move 2:

Notes:

Move Name:

Draw/sketch:

Prep Move 1:

Prep Move 2:

Notes:

Choreography notes

Cool down and stretch (10 min)

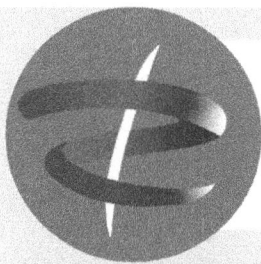

Self- Evaluation

Notes to improve on next time

Tricky move and the muscle groups to work on

Move Name: _____

Strengthen:

Stretch:

Other notes:

What tips helped me today?

Move Name: _____

Move Name: _____

Other: _____

Something that really clicked with me

Favourite or Inspiring music track

My Goal (something I look forward to)

I am proud of myself because...

Finding My Flow and Style

My favourite Floor combination is:

My favourite Spins to put together are:

Up the pole (or apparatus), I love to....

When Upside-down, I love doing this combination:

This is my preferred way to get myself Upside-down:

"You were born with wings, why prefer to crawl through life?"

-Rumi

Let's Review our Goal at the start...

Go back to page one... how are you going with your mini goals/steps? Are you on track?!

Review those steps- are they still what you feel is the pathway to your goal? Or would you like to update them?

Is your original goal still the same, or does it need updating?

My Ultimate Goal:

_____

_____

How it looks:

_____

_____

_____

_____

What it makes me feel like:

_____

_____

_____

_____

Steps to achieve that goal:

Steps (mini-goals)	Achieved by (date)	Completed date

By doing those unique, different things today, you are setting trends tomorrow. Creating a tomorrow where others can't do what you are doing, and may even aspire to do as you do!

Level: _____   Date: _____

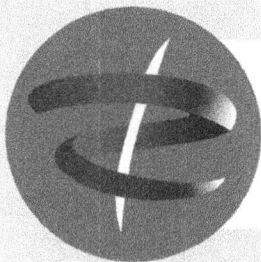

Training Record

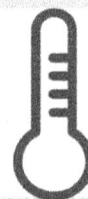

Colour in how stressed you are

Getting Started (10min)

Cardio Warm up:

Dynamic Stretches:

Conditioning:

Core Moves to work on today

Move Name:

Draw/sketch:

Prep Move 1:

Prep Move 2:

Notes:

Move Name:

Draw/sketch:

Prep Move 1:

Prep Move 2:

Notes:

Move Name:

Draw/sketch:

Prep Move 1:

Prep Move 2:

Notes:

Choreography notes

Cool down and stretch (10 min)

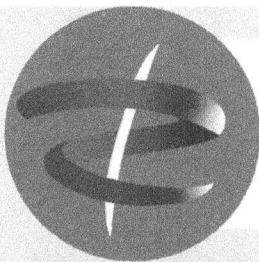

Self- Evaluation

Colour in how fatigued you are

Notes to improve on next time

Tricky move and the muscle groups to work on

Move Name: _____

Strengthen:

Stretch:

Other notes:

What tips helped me today?

Move Name: _____

Move Name: _____

Other: _____

Something that really clicked with me

Favourite or Inspiring music track

My Goal (something I look forward to)

I am proud of myself because...

Level: _____   Date: _____

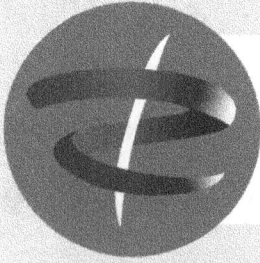

Training Record

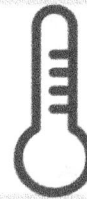

Colour in how stressed you are

Getting Started (10min)

Cardio Warm up:

Dynamic Stretches:

Conditioning:

Core Moves to work on today

Move Name:

Draw/sketch:

Prep Move 1:

Prep Move 2:

Notes:

Move Name:

Draw/sketch:

Prep Move 1:

Prep Move 2:

Notes:

Move Name:

Draw/sketch:

Prep Move 1:

Prep Move 2:

Notes:

Choreography notes

Cool down and stretch (10 min)

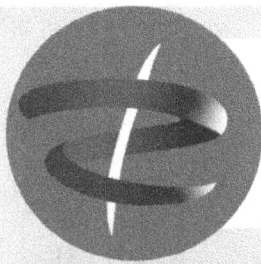

Self- Evaluation

Notes to improve on next time

Tricky move and the muscle groups to work on

Move Name: _____

Strengthen:

Stretch:

Other notes:

What tips helped me today?

Move Name: _____

Move Name: _____

Other: _____

Something that really clicked with me

Favourite or Inspiring music track

My Goal (something I look forward to)

I am proud of myself because...

Level: Date:

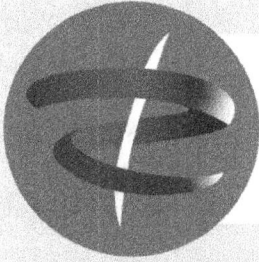

Training Record

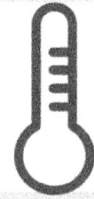

Colour in how stressed you are

Getting Started (10min)

Cardio Warm up:

Dynamic Stretches:

Conditioning:

Core Moves to work on today

Move Name:

Draw/sketch:

Prep Move 1:

Prep Move 2:

Notes:

Move Name:

Draw/sketch:

Prep Move 1:

Prep Move 2:

Notes:

Move Name:

Draw/sketch:

Prep Move 1:

Prep Move 2:

Notes:

Choreography notes

Cool down and stretch (10 min)

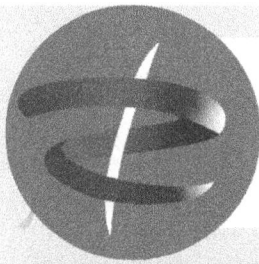

Self- Evaluation

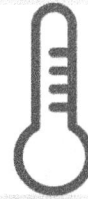

Colour in how fatigued you are

Notes to improve on next time

Tricky move and the muscle groups to work on

Move Name: _____

Strengthen:

Stretch:

Other notes:

What tips helped me today?

Move Name: _____

Move Name: _____

Other: _____

Something that really clicked with me

Favourite or Inspiring music track

My Goal (something I look forward to)

I am proud of myself because...

Level: Date:

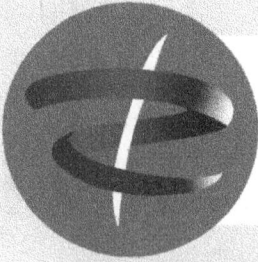

Training Record

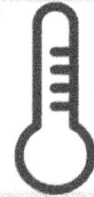

Colour in how stressed you are

Getting Started (10min)

Cardio Warm up:

Dynamic Stretches:

Conditioning:

Core Moves to work on today

Move Name:
Draw/sketch:

Prep Move 1:

Prep Move 2:

Notes:

Move Name:
Draw/sketch:

Prep Move 1:

Prep Move 2:

Notes:

Move Name:
Draw/sketch:

Prep Move 1:

Prep Move 2:

Notes:

Choreography notes

Cool down and stretch (10 min)

Personal Pole and Aerial Record   Rapture Arts

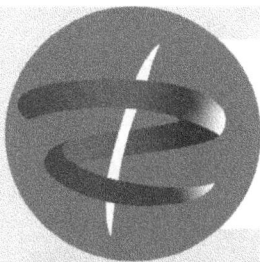

Self- Evaluation

Notes to improve on next time

Tricky move and the muscle groups to work on

Move Name: _____

Strengthen:

Stretch:

Other notes:

What tips helped me today?

Move Name: _____

Move Name: _____

Other: _____

Something that really clicked with me

Favourite or Inspiring music track

My Goal (something I look forward to)

I am proud of myself because...

Date Goal Set: Level:

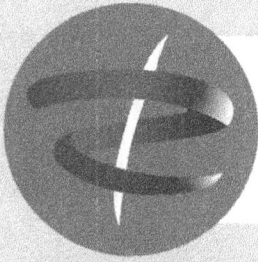

Strength Goals

What it will look like when I have achieved my goal.

Muscles required to condition or stretch for this to happen?

Strengthen:

Stretch:

Conditioning and flexibility drills, reps and requirements

Remember to maintain balance, remember you have a right and left side, as well as front and back. balance your training, not only in your body, but in relation to strength and flexibility.

Time Frame

Training how many days a week:

For how long?

Goal is to by achieved by:

Mini Goals that help with my big goal

Things I need to be able to achieve to reach my goal:

Notes

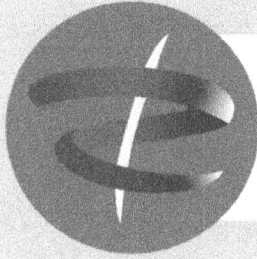

Strength Workout Planner

Warm Up

Training Drill (strength or flex)

Remember, it is not just about strength, it is also about ensuring your muscles are balanced, left and right, front and back. Also ensuring you stretch, not just strength train.

Reps

How many repetitions of the move

Sets

How many times we do the group of exercises

Cool Down

Level: Date:

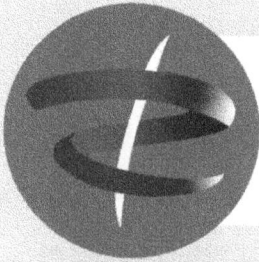

Training Record

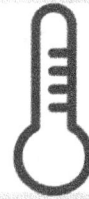

Colour in how stressed you are

Getting Started (10min)

Cardio Warm up:

Dynamic Stretches:

Conditioning:

Core Moves to work on today

Move Name:

Draw/sketch:

Prep Move 1:

Prep Move 2:

Notes:

Move Name:

Draw/sketch:

Prep Move 1:

Prep Move 2:

Notes:

Move Name:

Draw/sketch:

Prep Move 1:

Prep Move 2:

Notes:

Choreography notes

Cool down and stretch (10 min)

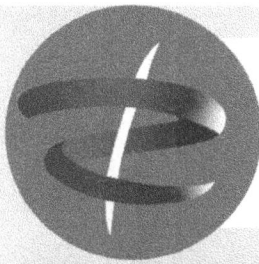

Self- Evaluation

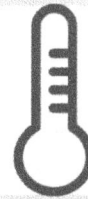

Notes to improve on next time

Tricky move and the muscle groups to work on

Move Name: _____

Strengthen:

Stretch:

Other notes:

What tips helped me today?

Move Name: _____

Move Name: _____

Other: _____

Something that really clicked with me

Favourite or Inspiring music track

My Goal (something I look forward to)

I am proud of myself because...

Level: Date:

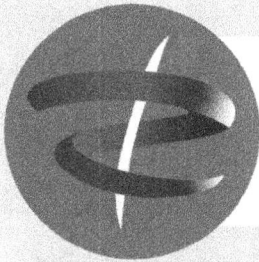

Training Record

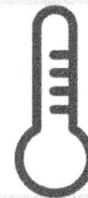

Colour in how stressed you are

Getting Started (10min)

Cardio Warm up: Dynamic Stretches: Conditioning:

Core Moves to work on today

Move Name: Move Name: Move Name:

Draw/sketch: Draw/sketch: Draw/sketch:

Prep Move 1:   Prep Move 1:   Prep Move 1:

Prep Move 2:   Prep Move 2:   Prep Move 2:

Notes: Notes: Notes:

Choreography notes

Cool down and stretch (10 min)

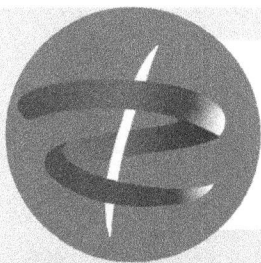

Self- Evaluation

Colour in how fatigued you are

Notes to improve on next time

Tricky move and the muscle groups to work on

Move Name: _____

Strengthen:

Stretch:

Other notes:

What tips helped me today?

Move Name: _____

Move Name: _____

Other: _____

Something that really clicked with me

Favourite or Inspiring music track

My Goal (something I look forward to)

I am proud of myself because...

Level: Date:

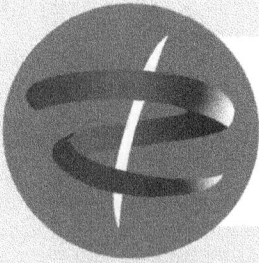

Training Record

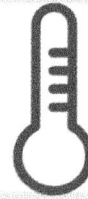

Colour in how stressed you are

Getting Started (10min)

Cardio Warm up:

Dynamic Stretches:

Conditioning:

Core Moves to work on today

Move Name:

Draw/sketch:

Prep Move 1:

Prep Move 2:

Notes:

Move Name:

Draw/sketch:

Prep Move 1:

Prep Move 2:

Notes:

Move Name:

Draw/sketch:

Prep Move 1:

Prep Move 2:

Notes:

Choreography notes

Cool down and stretch (10 min)

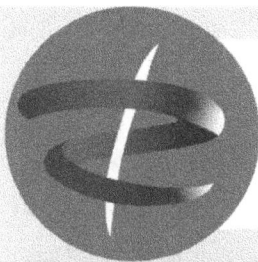

Self- Evaluation

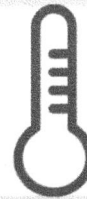

Notes to improve on next time

Tricky move and the muscle groups to work on

Move Name: _____

Strengthen:

Stretch:

Other notes:

What tips helped me today?

Move Name: _____

Move Name: _____

Other: _____

Something that really clicked with me

Favourite or Inspiring music track

My Goal (something I look forward to)

I am proud of myself because...

Level: Date:

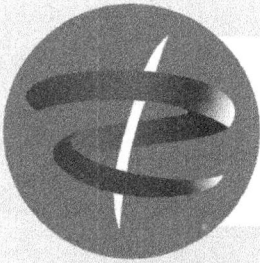

Training Record

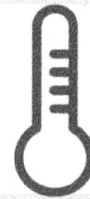

Colour in how stressed you are

Getting Started (10min)

Cardio Warm up:

Dynamic Stretches:

Conditioning:

Core Moves to work on today

Move Name:

Draw/sketch:

Prep Move 1:

Prep Move 2:

Notes:

Move Name:

Draw/sketch:

Prep Move 1:

Prep Move 2:

Notes:

Move Name:

Draw/sketch:

Prep Move 1:

Prep Move 2:

Notes:

Choreography notes

Cool down and stretch (10 min)

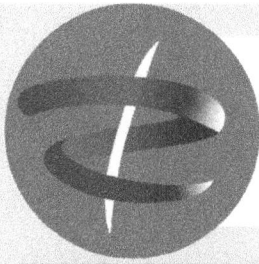

Self- Evaluation

Notes to improve on next time

Tricky move and the muscle groups to work on

Move Name: _____

Strengthen:

Stretch:

Other notes:

What tips helped me today?

Move Name: _____

Move Name: _____

Other: _____

Something that really clicked with me

Favourite or Inspiring music track

My Goal (something I look forward to)

I am proud of myself because...

Steps to Success!

Believe in your goal and in yourself!!!

If you don't believe, then you are stuck here. What do you need to do to believe? Do you need to see it? Plan it? Goal Set? Vision Board? Break it down to make smaller, more manageable steps? Track your progress so you can see it? Get a training buddy you have faith in and do it together to get yourselves motivated?

Be Clear about what your goal is.

What is it? Is it a move, a competition, a flow? How does it look, how does it feel? Do you want to achieve "x" number of push-ups or hold a move for "x" long? To "pole dance" isn't clarity... to be able to achieve x move with ease is clarity... or to be able to enter in the "x" amateur competition in 9 months' time... is clarity... be clear, simple, straight forward and specific with your goal.

Commit to your goal - is that a certain time or space?

This differs depending on your goal! Create a promise to yourself, steps to make your goal realistic. Do you need to spend 45 minutes every third day training a particular move, with stretching and conditioning focused on other days? Do you need to do 25 push-ups daily? Break down your goal, choreograph 20 seconds of a routine every Monday, and train that 20 seconds for the rest of the week before adding to it the following Monday... What specific time frame or amount or space are you going to set aside each day to make your goal a reality.

Arm yourself with the knowledge to be able to achieve your goal.

Where do you need to go to learn what you need to learn? Who inspires you or teaches in a way that helps you learn? What book do you need to read, or tutorial do you need to watch? What Pole Fitness School do you need to attend? Do you need to learn about Pole, about circus aerials, about music, about costuming, flexibility or fitness? – what do you need and where can you go to help you?

Stop putting it off... create your plan... and get to it!

Someone who doesn't give up, constantly progresses. Without doing the same, you won't beat them!

Design your Costume

Visualization is key to being able to think positive and see your success. So, depending on your goal, putting your costume down on paper may be the next step in your visual journey... if it doesn't relate to your goal, it can still be a bit of fun!

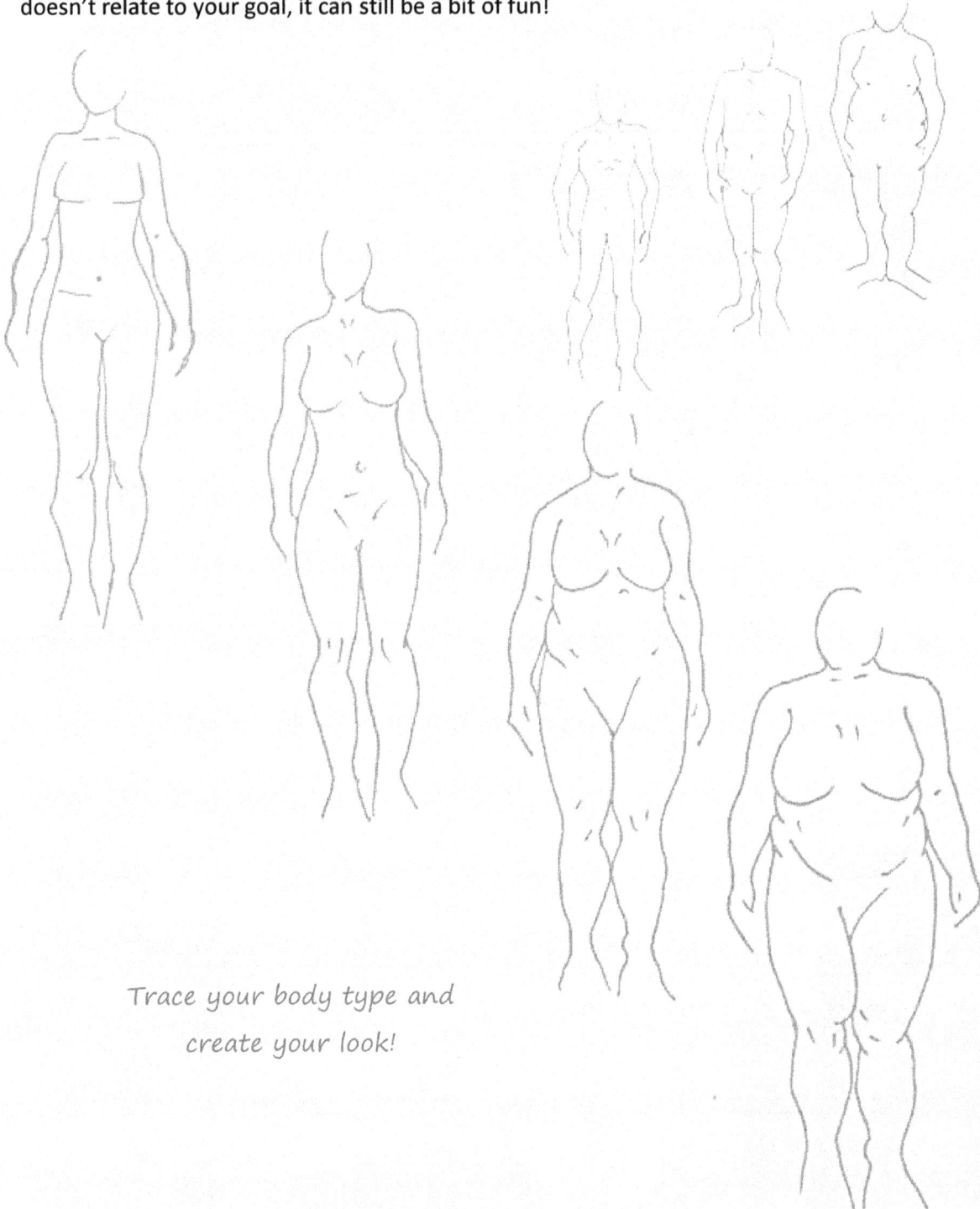

Trace your body type and
create your look!

Create yourself, don't waste your time trying to find yourself!

Planning your Performing Persona and Character Image

Stage Name:

Any important back story:

Mood and style of performance:

Era (if applicable):

Song/s, their meaning and their genre:

Costuming Style:

Comfort/Movement and grip point requirements:

Colours:

Fabric requirements:

Other:

Hair and make-up requirements/notes:

Props and accessories:

What about Make-Up?

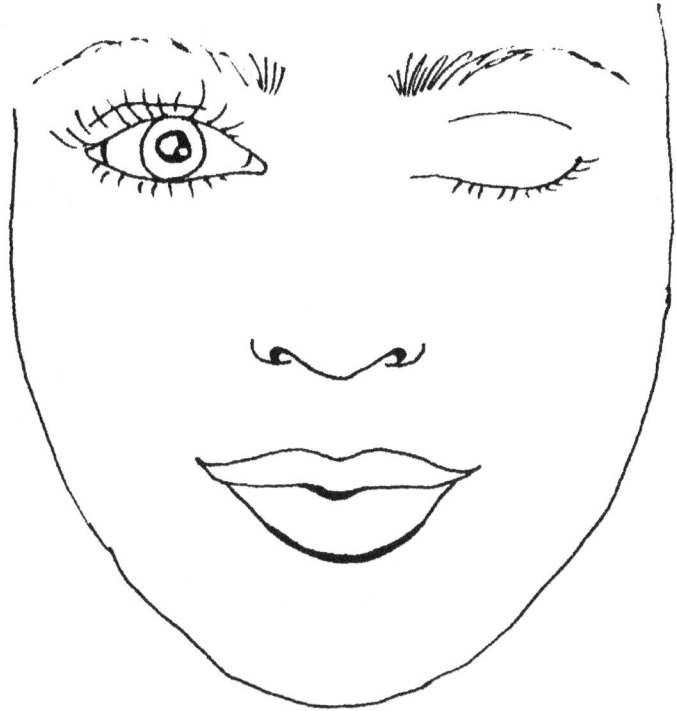

Eyes:

Eye Brows:

Eye Shadow:

      Base Colour:

      Crease:

      Outer Corner:

      Inner Corner:

Eye Liner:

Lower Lash-line:

Mascara:

Lashes/lash style:

Other special notes:

Face:

Primer:

Concealer:

Foundation:

Powder:

Blush:

Bronzer:

Contour:

Highlight:

Setting Spray:

Glitter/Gems/Accessories:

Facial Hair:

Face/Body Paint:

Other notes:

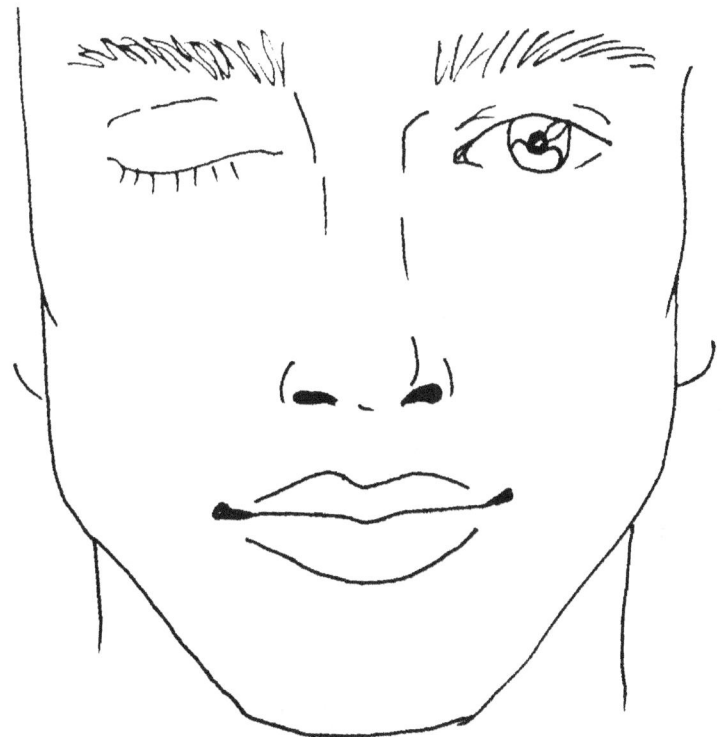

Lips:

Liner:

Gloss:

Colour:

Lipstick:

Era Specific: *Era:*

Lip Shape:

Blush style/location:

Eye-liner style:

Hair-style:

Level: _____   Date: _____

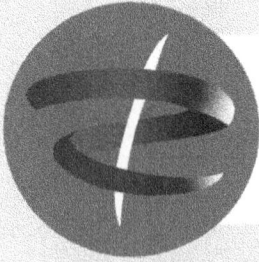

Training Record

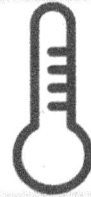

Colour in how stressed you are

Getting Started (10min)

Cardio Warm up:

Dynamic Stretches:

Conditioning:

Core Moves to work on today

Move Name:
Draw/sketch:

Prep Move 1:

Prep Move 2:

Notes:

Move Name:
Draw/sketch:

Prep Move 1:

Prep Move 2:

Notes:

Move Name:
Draw/sketch:

Prep Move 1:

Prep Move 2:

Notes:

Choreography notes

Cool down and stretch (10 min)

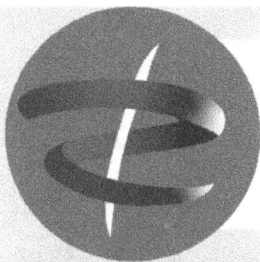

Self- Evaluation

Colour in how fatigued you are

Notes to improve on next time

Tricky move and the muscle groups to work on

Move Name: _____

Strengthen:

Stretch:

Other notes:

What tips helped me today?

Move Name: _____

Move Name: _____

Other: _____

Something that really clicked with me

Favourite or Inspiring music track

My Goal (something I look forward to)

I am proud of myself because...

Level: _____   Date: _____

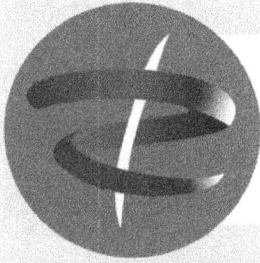

Training Record

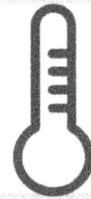

Getting Started (10min)

Cardio Warm up:

Dynamic Stretches:

Conditioning:

Core Moves to work on today

Move Name:

Draw/sketch:

Prep Move 1:

Prep Move 2:

Notes:

Move Name:

Draw/sketch:

Prep Move 1:

Prep Move 2:

Notes:

Move Name:

Draw/sketch:

Prep Move 1:

Prep Move 2:

Notes:

Choreography notes

Cool down and stretch (10 min)

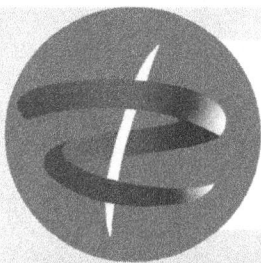

Self- Evaluation

Colour in how fatigued you are

Notes to improve on next time

Tricky move and the muscle groups to work on

Move Name: _____

Strengthen:

Stretch:

Other notes:

What tips helped me today?

Move Name: _____

Move Name: _____

Other: _____

Something that really clicked with me

Favourite or Inspiring music track

My Goal (something I look forward to)

I am proud of myself because...

Level: _____   Date: _____

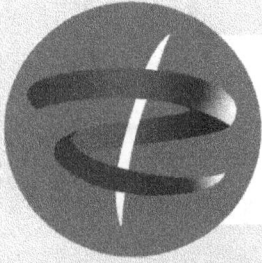

Training Record

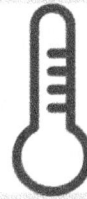

Colour in how stressed you are

Getting Started (10min)

Cardio Warm up:

Dynamic Stretches:

Conditioning:

Core Moves to work on today

Move Name:

Draw/sketch:

Prep Move 1:

Prep Move 2:

Notes:

Move Name:

Draw/sketch:

Prep Move 1:

Prep Move 2:

Notes:

Move Name:

Draw/sketch:

Prep Move 1:

Prep Move 2:

Notes:

Choreography notes

Cool down and stretch (10 min)

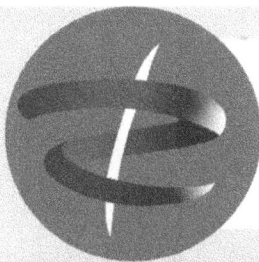

Self- Evaluation

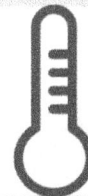

Colour in how fatigued you are

Notes to improve on next time

Tricky move and the muscle groups to work on

Move Name: _____

Strengthen:

Stretch:

Other notes:

What tips helped me today?

Move Name: _____

Move Name: _____

Other: _____

Something that really clicked with me

Favourite or Inspiring music track

My Goal (something I look forward to)

I am proud of myself because...

Level: _____   Date: _____

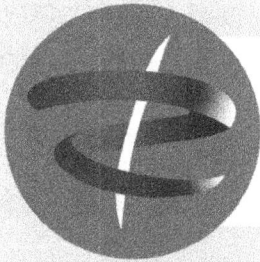

Training Record

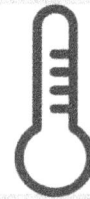

Colour in how stressed you are

Getting Started (10min)

Cardio Warm up:

Dynamic Stretches:

Conditioning:

Core Moves to work on today

Move Name:

Draw/sketch:

Prep Move 1:

Prep Move 2:

Notes:

Move Name:

Draw/sketch:

Prep Move 1:

Prep Move 2:

Notes:

Move Name:

Draw/sketch:

Prep Move 1:

Prep Move 2:

Notes:

Choreography notes

Cool down and stretch (10 min)

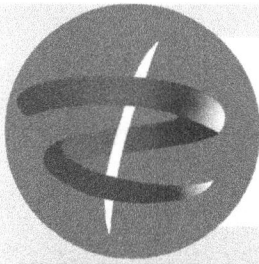

Self- Evaluation

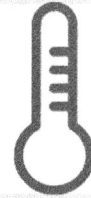

Notes to improve on next time

Tricky move and the muscle groups to work on

Move Name: _____

Strengthen:

Stretch:

Other notes:

What tips helped me today?

Move Name: _____

Move Name: _____

Other: _____

Something that really clicked with me

Favourite or Inspiring music track

My Goal (something I look forward to)

I am proud of myself because...

Transitions! *(Pole focused but still important for Aerials)*

Transitions are so important, transitioning smoothly is a great habit as it makes you focus on the next step and not dropping out of moves, thus protecting yourself from potential injury. It is also a great way to find your flow and your unique style. Transitions are the key to a magical performance! Finding new transitions also expands your understanding of the moves themselves.

Knowing your move and your flow helps heaps. As you grow your experience and understanding in pole fitness, it becomes less conscious as to where to place your leg, in say an outside leg hang, and how the grip feels... in the beginning, that requires a lot of thought to ensure you're safe. One of the things that helps this become more natural is understanding the move. Comfort and understanding of the grip and body placement. What muscles do you need to focus on- this is such an integral understanding, instead of saying I can't do this, knowing what muscles you are supposed to be activating, allows you to know what muscle groups to strengthen or stretch in order to achieve the move. Alternatively, it allows you to realise that you were activating your upper body, instead of your core, and that may be the key to achieving the move.

Once you understand the move, you can look at your contact points with the pole, what is your main supporting grip point, and where is your centre of gravity? These are vital pointers when looking at intricate advanced transitions from one move to another. Moving from one pole position into another pole position is an art, now to do that without interrupting your momentum from the pole move is where the flow really comes into it. This is so much more effective when your grips and body positions share a common point of contact with the pole.

Fav pole move	Points of contact with the pole	Muscle groups activated in this move	Transition idea or pole move to transition into	New pole moves points of contact with the pole

"Most obstacles melt away when we make up our minds to walk boldly through them."

-Orison Swett Marden

Dream it, imagine it, you can do it!

**When I started;
this move seemed impossible!!**

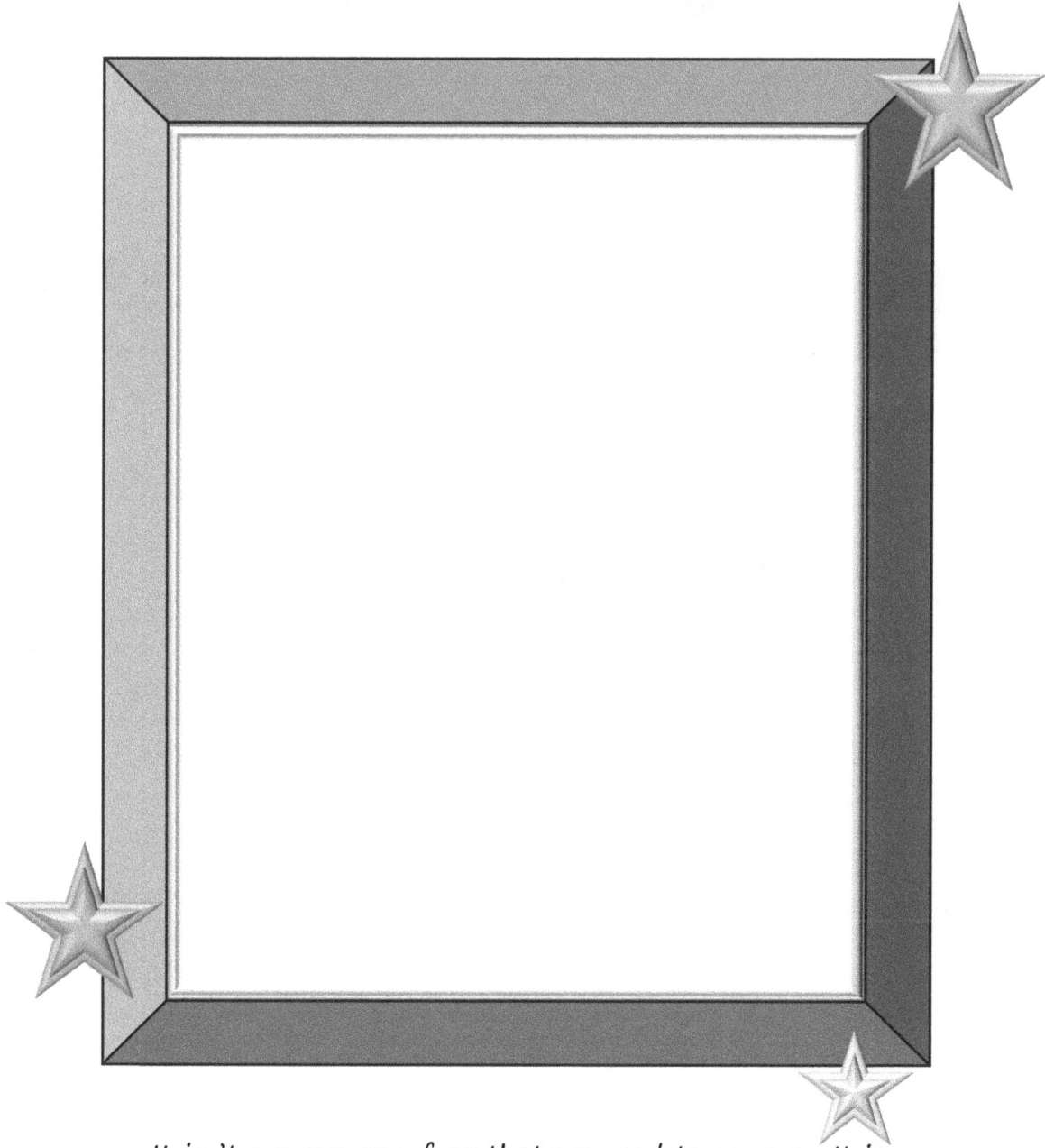

It isn't a move or a fear that we need to conquer. It is ourselves!

Level: Date:

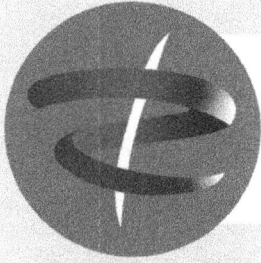

Training Record

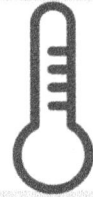

Colour in how stressed you are

Getting Started (10min)

Cardio Warm up:

Dynamic Stretches:

Conditioning:

Core Moves to work on today

Move Name:

Draw/sketch:

Prep Move 1:

Prep Move 2:

Notes:

Move Name:

Draw/sketch:

Prep Move 1:

Prep Move 2:

Notes:

Move Name:

Draw/sketch:

Prep Move 1:

Prep Move 2:

Notes:

Choreography notes

Cool down and stretch (10 min)

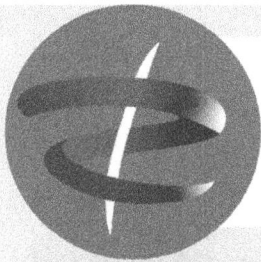

Self- Evaluation

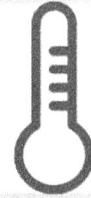

Colour in how fatigued you are

Notes to improve on next time

Tricky move and the muscle groups to work on

Move Name: _____

Strengthen:

Stretch:

Other notes:

What tips helped me today?

Move Name: _____

Move Name: _____

Other: _____

Something that really clicked with me

Favourite or Inspiring music track

My Goal (something I look forward to)

I am proud of myself because...

Level: Date:

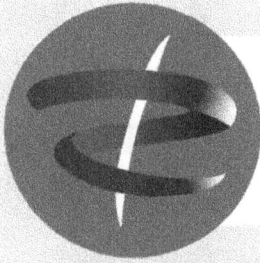

Training Record

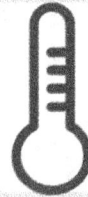

Colour in how stressed you are

Getting Started (10min)

Cardio Warm up:

Dynamic Stretches:

Conditioning:

Core Moves to work on today

Move Name:

Draw/sketch:

Prep Move 1:

Prep Move 2:

Notes:

Move Name:

Draw/sketch:

Prep Move 1:

Prep Move 2:

Notes:

Move Name:

Draw/sketch:

Prep Move 1:

Prep Move 2:

Notes:

Choreography notes

Cool down and stretch (10 min)

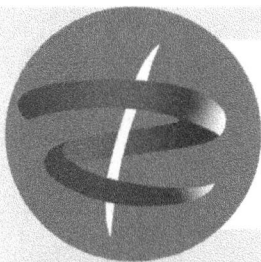

Self- Evaluation

Colour in how fatigued you are

Notes to improve on next time

Tricky move and the muscle groups to work on

Move Name: _____

Strengthen:

Stretch:

Other notes:

What tips helped me today?

Move Name: _____

Move Name: _____

Other: _____

Something that really clicked with me

Favourite or Inspiring music track

My Goal (something I look forward to)

I am proud of myself because...

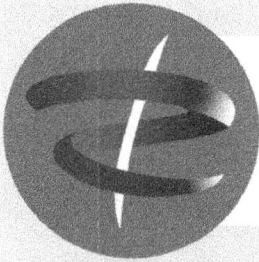

Training Record

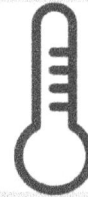

Colour in how stressed you are

Getting Started (10min)

Cardio Warm up:

Dynamic Stretches:

Conditioning:

Core Moves to work on today

Move Name:

Draw/sketch:

Prep Move 1:

Prep Move 2:

Notes:

Move Name:

Draw/sketch:

Prep Move 1:

Prep Move 2:

Notes:

Move Name:

Draw/sketch:

Prep Move 1:

Prep Move 2:

Notes:

Choreography notes

Cool down and stretch (10 min)

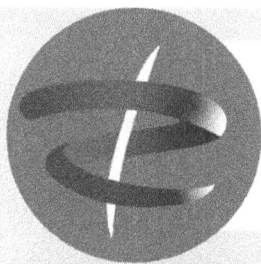

Self- Evaluation

Colour in how fatigued you are

Notes to improve on next time

Tricky move and the muscle groups to work on

Move Name: _____

Strengthen:

Stretch:

Other notes:

What tips helped me today?

Move Name: _____

Move Name: _____

Other: _____

Something that really clicked with me

Favourite or Inspiring music track

My Goal (something I look forward to)

I am proud of myself because...

Level: Date:

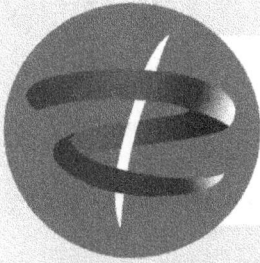

Training Record

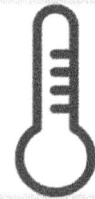

Colour in how stressed you are

Getting Started (10min)

Cardio Warm up:

Dynamic Stretches:

Conditioning:

Core Moves to work on today

Move Name:

Draw/sketch:

Prep Move 1:

Prep Move 2:

Notes:

Move Name:

Draw/sketch:

Prep Move 1:

Prep Move 2:

Notes:

Move Name:

Draw/sketch:

Prep Move 1:

Prep Move 2:

Notes:

Choreography notes

Cool down and stretch (10 min)

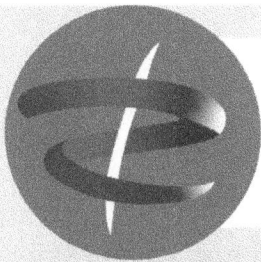

Self- Evaluation

Notes to improve on next time

Tricky move and the muscle groups to work on

Move Name: _____

Strengthen:

Stretch:

Other notes:

What tips helped me today?

Move Name: _____

Move Name: _____

Other: _____

Something that really clicked with me

Favourite or Inspiring music track

My Goal (something I look forward to)

I am proud of myself because...

Home training can be daunting, especially if you don't have a pole. But there are always options of things to work on, consider or visualize at home to assist with your pole training. Please be aware of the risks of not having someone there to spot or correct techniques and assist you. Only perform training exercises that you are comfortable with and have an understanding of the technique and risks of performing such movements.

RAPTURE
Arts
MOVE POINTERS

MY GOAL MOVE

POINTERS TO WORK ON

OFF THE POLE OPTIONS

#RaptureArts

Things to do to still feel productive on your rest day

A rest day doesn't mean to be completely sedentary. As much as you want to rest, you still want to remain active in your daily routine. The most important thing is to listen to your body. What is it that your body needs? We know we need to ensure we have enough sleep, that we eat healthily, and keep hydrated. But if your body needs that warm bath to relax the muscles, a stretch, or a light walk to keep things moving, then listen! Rest days are important, not just for your body to get the chance to rest and recover, but for your mind to have that space too. Remember to continue making progress. You need this!

So, what can you do for your body on these days?
- Go for a gentle swim
- Have a light stroll
- Stretch or foam roll out your muscles
- Grab a massage, and treat yourself a little!
- Some yoga can help if you aren't going too intense all week.

Remember, this is only if your body is up for it and asking for it. Rest days help your muscles repair from all their work during the week. They give your immune system a chance to recover too, as getting too worn out can weaken your immune system. Whether that is worn out from physical training or mental stress, it takes its toll eventually. Rest days are a great way of keeping on top. You can even use these days as your planning day, to plan your week's goals and training. Look at your progress from your last goals, and renew your focus. That way, you still feel like you are being productive, even if you are having a complete rest and relaxation day with no training. What you eat also affects your recovery, so it isn't a rest day from eating right. In fact, you can even use your rest day to meal prep whilst also prepping your week's training!

You can even look at other skills; it could be finding inspiration for combinations to work on during the week, observing others' shows, training and routines for inspiration. Or finding a rest day hobby, something less intense that still works your mind, juggling, for example, works your hand-eye coordination, as well as your mind; coordination in poi is a little bit more in the shoulders in a different way, so could be on a less active day, even hula hooping is great. These are all active, without being intense, so they are things you can use on a lesser training day or an active recovery day.

All that sounds like work, so ensure you get one rest day that is exactly that, rest!! Spend time with the family, catch up with friends, and don't let the world get on top of you with work, work, work- spend a day for you! Whether that be social or a day to have a bath and do your nails. What is it that you need? A day like this helps you keep on top of things, which then assists with your training, so don't feel guilty for taking a day. Enjoy it! Have an early night, and come back rejuvenated and ready for the week ahead!
Listen to your body, and allow it the time it needs.

Note: if you have any corrective or rehabilitation exercises, ensure that you perform these as per a medical professional's advice.

Level: Date:

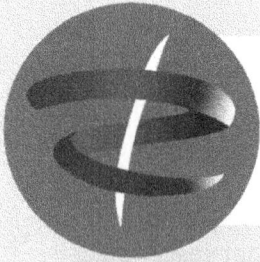

Training Record

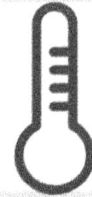

Colour in how stressed you are

Getting Started (10min)

Cardio Warm up:

Dynamic Stretches:

Conditioning:

Core Moves to work on today

Move Name:

Draw/sketch:

Prep Move 1:

Prep Move 2:

Notes:

Move Name:

Draw/sketch:

Prep Move 1:

Prep Move 2:

Notes:

Move Name:

Draw/sketch:

Prep Move 1:

Prep Move 2:

Notes:

Choreography notes

Cool down and stretch (10 min)

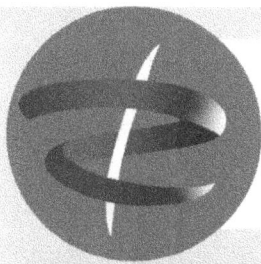

Self- Evaluation

Notes to improve on next time

Tricky move and the muscle groups to work on

Move Name: _____

Strengthen:

Stretch:

Other notes:

What tips helped me today?

Move Name: _____

Move Name: _____

Other: _____

Something that really clicked with me

Favourite or Inspiring music track

My Goal (something I look forward to)

I am proud of myself because...

Level: Date:

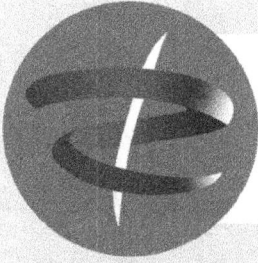

Training Record

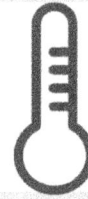

Colour in how stressed you are

Getting Started (10min)

Cardio Warm up:

Dynamic Stretches:

Conditioning:

Core Moves to work on today

Move Name:

Draw/sketch:

Prep Move 1:

Prep Move 2:

Notes:

Move Name:

Draw/sketch:

Prep Move 1:

Prep Move 2:

Notes:

Move Name:

Draw/sketch:

Prep Move 1:

Prep Move 2:

Notes:

Choreography notes

Cool down and stretch (10 min)

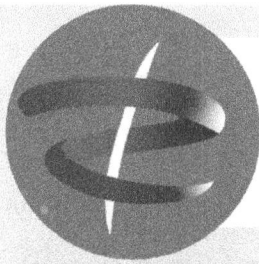

Self- Evaluation

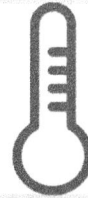

Colour in how fatigued you are

Notes to improve on next time

Tricky move and the muscle groups to work on

Move Name: _____

Strengthen:

Stretch:

Other notes:

What tips helped me today?

Move Name: _____

Move Name: _____

Other: _____

Something that really clicked with me

Favourite or Inspiring music track

My Goal (something I look forward to)

I am proud of myself because...

Level: Date:

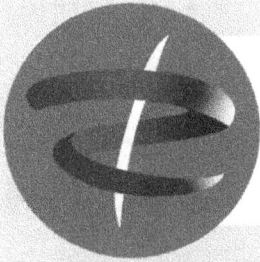

Training Record

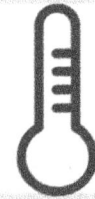

Colour in how stressed you are

Getting Started (10min)

Cardio Warm up:

Dynamic Stretches:

Conditioning:

Core Moves to work on today

Move Name:

Draw/sketch:

Prep Move 1:

Prep Move 2:

Notes:

Move Name:

Draw/sketch:

Prep Move 1:

Prep Move 2:

Notes:

Move Name:

Draw/sketch:

Prep Move 1:

Prep Move 2:

Notes:

Choreography notes

Cool down and stretch (10 min)

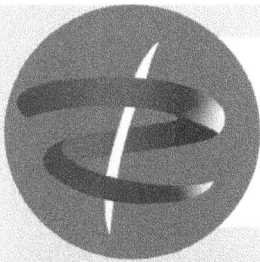

Self- Evaluation

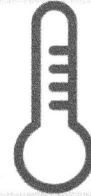

Colour in how fatigued you are

Notes to improve on next time

Tricky move and the muscle groups to work on

Move Name: _____

Strengthen:

Stretch:

Other notes:

What tips helped me today?

Move Name: _____

Move Name: _____

Other: _____

Something that really clicked with me

Favourite or Inspiring music track

My Goal (something I look forward to)

I am proud of myself because...

Level: _____   Date: _____

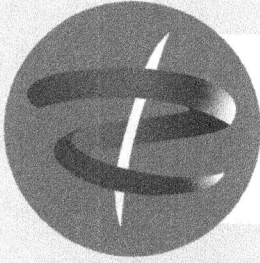

Training Record

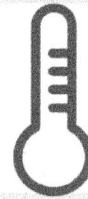

Colour in how stressed you are

Getting Started (10min)

Cardio Warm up:

Dynamic Stretches:

Conditioning:

Core Moves to work on today

Move Name:

Draw/sketch:

Prep Move 1:

Prep Move 2:

Notes:

Move Name:

Draw/sketch:

Prep Move 1:

Prep Move 2:

Notes:

Move Name:

Draw/sketch:

Prep Move 1:

Prep Move 2:

Notes:

Choreography notes

Cool down and stretch (10 min)

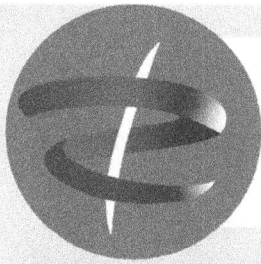

Self- Evaluation

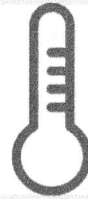

Colour in how fatigued you are

Notes to improve on next time

Tricky move and the muscle groups to work on

Move Name: _____

Strengthen:

Stretch:

Other notes:

What tips helped me today?

Move Name: _____

Move Name: _____

Other: _____

Something that really clicked with me

Favourite or Inspiring music track

My Goal (something I look forward to)

I am proud of myself because...

Why does everyone talk about needing to drink water?

Hydration is vital when training, it is pretty much the key to optimizing your performance when training. I know you have heard it all before, but it isn't just so you don't get heat stroke and pass out, or because it is "healthy" … there are other reasons too! Have you ever wondered what drinking water does when you exercise?

- It helps stop you from overheating! Yes, just like a puppy pants after exercise to maintain body temperature and cool down. We drink water!
- Keeping hydrated actually helps with muscle cramps. It also helps the body move fluids with important stuff in it, to the muscles, as well as toxins away from the muscles. So, it can help recovery after training! (When you train, your muscles get little "tears", not the big, scary, ouchy ones, but little ones to assist with muscle growth. These "tears" need to recover and help to build the muscle, which requires us to be hydrated… we also want to flush some of the lactic acid away to help us recover quicker!)
- Your alertness starts to waver if you are dehydrated, and thus your performance is affected. You may feel like you can do things still, but potentially not to the standard or level that you normally do.
- Maintains the balance of fluid in your body, as you are sweating some of it out! (Fluid in your body helps with so much, from taking nutrients to cells, flushing away toxins, reducing muscle fatigue, keeping the skin hydrated, and that is without touching on bowel function, circulation, and reduction on inflammation and all these amazing things your body can do!)

Remember, the amount of water that you need to drink is based on a number of factors, not just the intensity of your workout, or how long you have worked out for, but also things like heat and humidity, and your personal sweat rate!

Signs that you may be dehydrated

- Muscle cramps
- High pulse rate
- Being lightheaded or dizzy
- Nausea
- Low energy
- Potential headache
- Even tiredness and having a dry mouth can be mild symptoms

If you have done a long or a high-intensity work out consider low sugar options to provide your muscles with vitamins and nutrients, and thus energy. Things with potassium and electrolytes can help you to train for a bit longer, or help you in recovery after training. You can make some really nice homemade electrolyte drinks too, using things like cucumber lime and coconut water, or orange and lemon juice with some salt, honey, and water. Have a look around for a recipe that suits you!

Remember, you must drink water, before, during, and after exercise. The amount depends on your body, environment, and training regime. Remember to listen to your body and stop and rest when needed.

Move Name: **Level:**

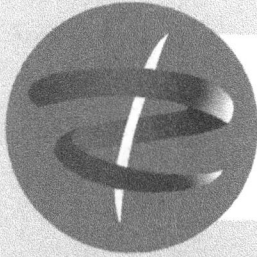

Move Goals

Picture of Move

Steps on how to get into the move.

Progress notes and tips

Conditioning and Flexibility needed

Transition into move

Achieved on my:
Right Side? ☐   Left side? ☐

Transition out of move

Achieved on my:
Right Side? ☐   Left side? ☐

Move Regressions

Move Progressions

Level: _____   Date: _____

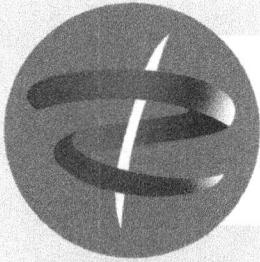

Training Record

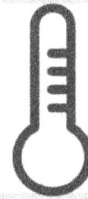

Colour in how stressed you are

Getting Started (10min)

Cardio Warm up:

Dynamic Stretches:

Conditioning:

Core Moves to work on today

Move Name:
Draw/sketch:

Prep Move 1:

Prep Move 2:

Notes:

Move Name:
Draw/sketch:

Prep Move 1:

Prep Move 2:

Notes:

Move Name:
Draw/sketch:

Prep Move 1:

Prep Move 2:

Notes:

Choreography notes

Cool down and stretch (10 min)

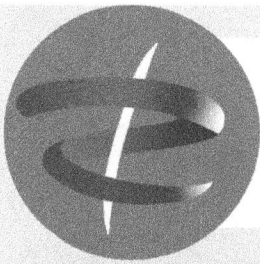

Self- Evaluation

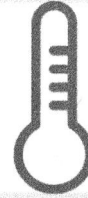

Colour in how fatigued you are

Notes to improve on next time

Tricky move and the muscle groups to work on

Move Name: _____

Strengthen:

Stretch:

Other notes:

What tips helped me today?

Move Name: _____

Move Name: _____

Other: _____

Something that really clicked with me

Favourite or Inspiring music track

My Goal (something I look forward to)

I am proud of myself because...

Level:	Date:

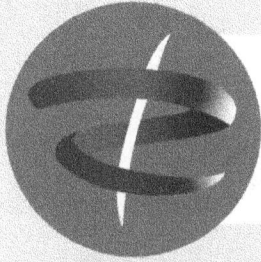

Training Record

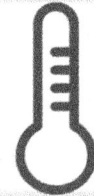

Colour in how stressed you are

Getting Started (10min)

Cardio Warm up:

Dynamic Stretches:

Conditioning:

Core Moves to work on today

Move Name:

Draw/sketch:

Prep Move 1:

Prep Move 2:

Notes:

Move Name:

Draw/sketch:

Prep Move 1:

Prep Move 2:

Notes:

Move Name:

Draw/sketch:

Prep Move 1:

Prep Move 2:

Notes:

Choreography notes

Cool down and stretch (10 min)

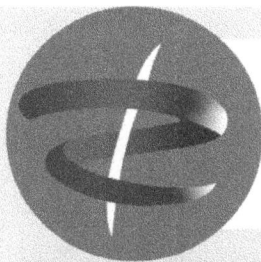

Self- Evaluation

Notes to improve on next time

Tricky move and the muscle groups to work on

Move Name: _____

Strengthen:

Stretch:

Other notes:

What tips helped me today?

Move Name: _____

Move Name: _____

Other: _____

Something that really clicked with me

Favourite or Inspiring music track

My Goal (something I look forward to)

I am proud of myself because...

Level:

Date:

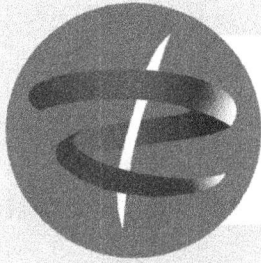

Training Record

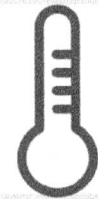

Colour in how stressed you are

Getting Started (10min)

Cardio Warm up:

Dynamic Stretches:

Conditioning:

Core Moves to work on today

Move Name:

Draw/sketch:

Prep Move 1:

Prep Move 2:

Notes:

Move Name:

Draw/sketch:

Prep Move 1:

Prep Move 2:

Notes:

Move Name:

Draw/sketch:

Prep Move 1:

Prep Move 2:

Notes:

Choreography notes

Cool down and stretch (10 min)

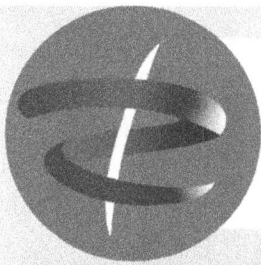

Self- Evaluation

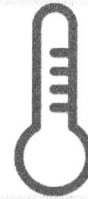

Colour in how fatigued you are

Notes to improve on next time

Tricky move and the muscle groups to work on

Move Name: _____

Strengthen:

Stretch:

Other notes:

What tips helped me today?

Move Name: _____

Move Name: _____

Other: _____

Something that really clicked with me

Favourite or Inspiring music track

My Goal (something I look forward to)

I am proud of myself because...

Level: Date:

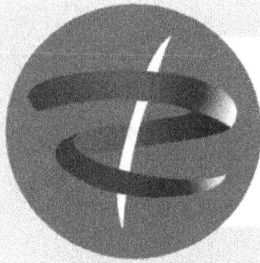

Training Record

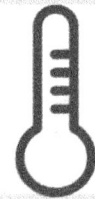

Colour in how stressed you are

Getting Started (10min)

Cardio Warm up:

Dynamic Stretches:

Conditioning:

Core Moves to work on today

Move Name:

Draw/sketch:

Prep Move 1:

Prep Move 2:

Notes:

Move Name:

Draw/sketch:

Prep Move 1:

Prep Move 2:

Notes:

Move Name:

Draw/sketch:

Prep Move 1:

Prep Move 2:

Notes:

Choreography notes

Cool down and stretch (10 min)

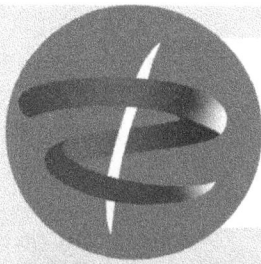

Self- Evaluation

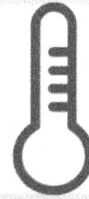

Colour in how fatigued you are

Notes to improve on next time

Tricky move and the muscle groups to work on

Move Name: _____

Strengthen:

Stretch:

Other notes:

What tips helped me today?

Move Name: _____

Move Name: _____

Other: _____

Something that really clicked with me

Favourite or Inspiring music track

My Goal (something I look forward to)

I am proud of myself because...

My Future Goals

Strength Goals

Goal	Steps	Achieve by (date)

Flexibility Goals

Goal	Steps	Achieve by (date)

Combination and Transition Goals

Goal	Steps	Achieve by (date)

The adventure has just begun!

Enjoy the ride and be in charge of your direction!